Where, Oh Where Tooth Fairy Go?

By Rachel Grider, RDH

Illustrated by Summer Morrison

This book belongs to:

_____

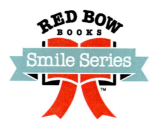

For Mags – R.G.
For my Dad – S.M.

Published by Red Bow Books LLC
The Smile Series

ISBN 978-1-7321568-1-4

Copyright © 2021 by Rachel Grider
Illustration © 2021 by Summer Morrison
All Rights Reserved

Printed in the Untied States of America

Library of Congress Control Number:
2020924959

This publication and all contents within may not be reproduced or transmitted in any part or in its entirety without the written permission of the author.

For more information, visit our website: www.RedBowBooks.com

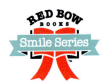

Making Little Smiles Brighter One Book at a Time!

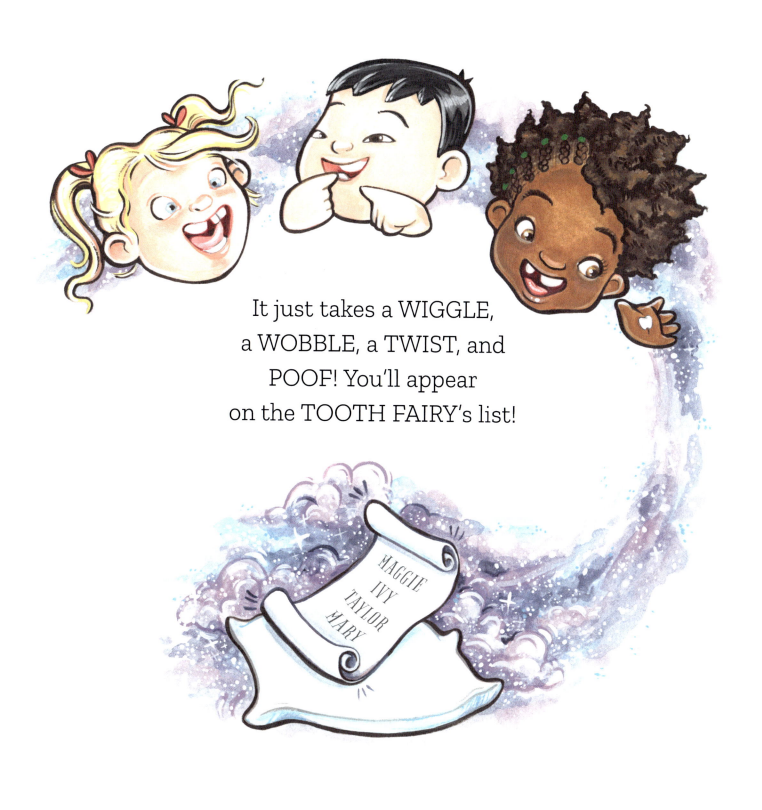

It just takes a WIGGLE, a WOBBLE, a TWIST, and POOF! You'll appear on the TOOTH FAIRY's list!

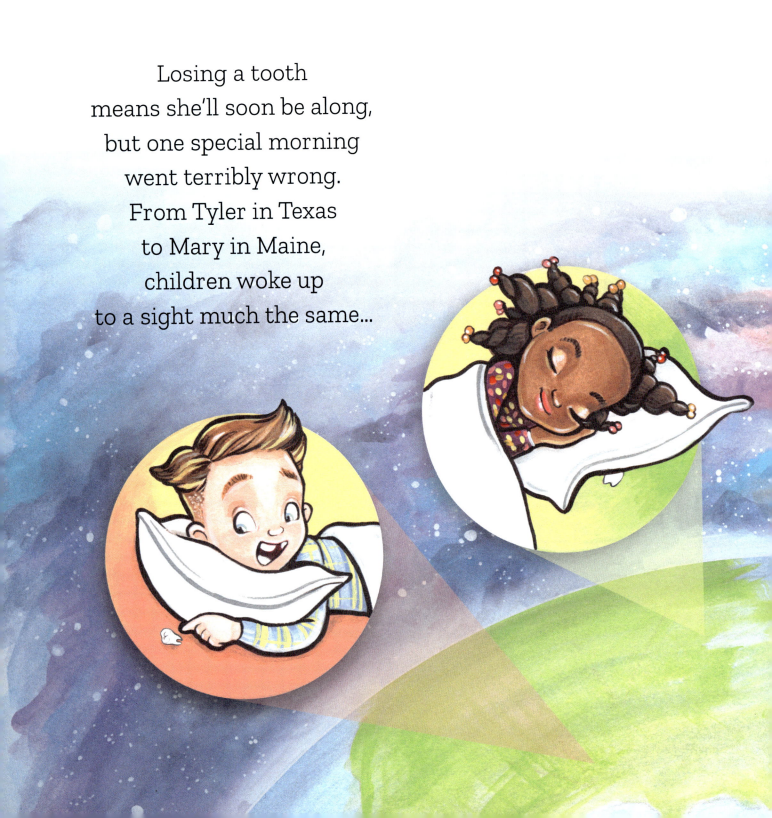

Losing a tooth
means she'll soon be along,
but one special morning
went terribly wrong.
From Tyler in Texas
to Mary in Maine,
children woke up
to a sight much the same...

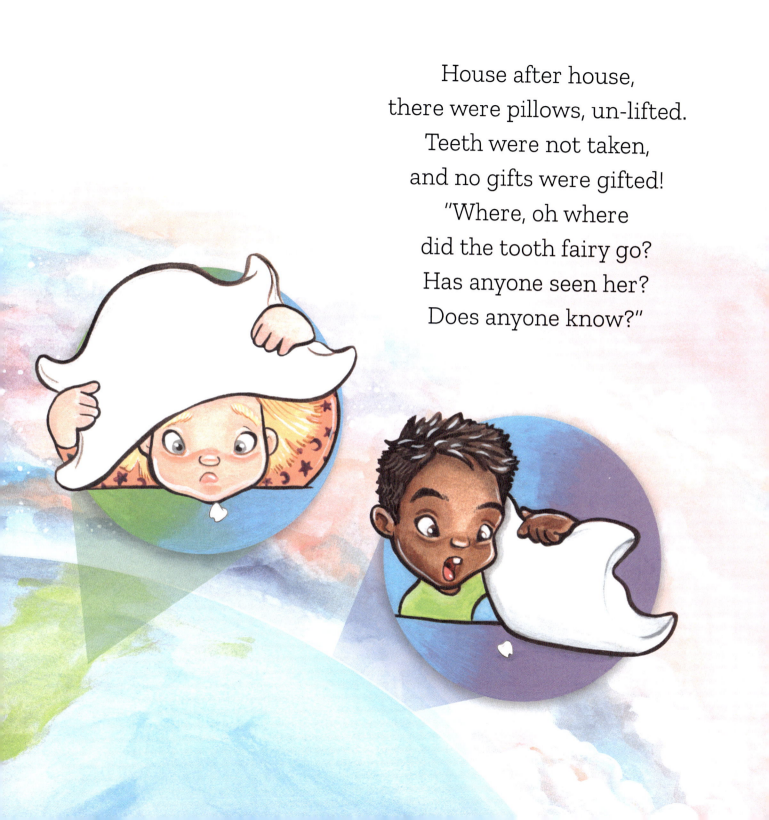

House after house,
there were pillows, un-lifted.
Teeth were not taken,
and no gifts were gifted!
"Where, oh where
did the tooth fairy go?
Has anyone seen her?
Does anyone know?"

Children set out.
They searched high and low,
but no one could find her.
Where did she go???

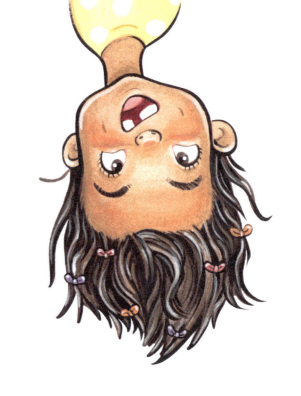
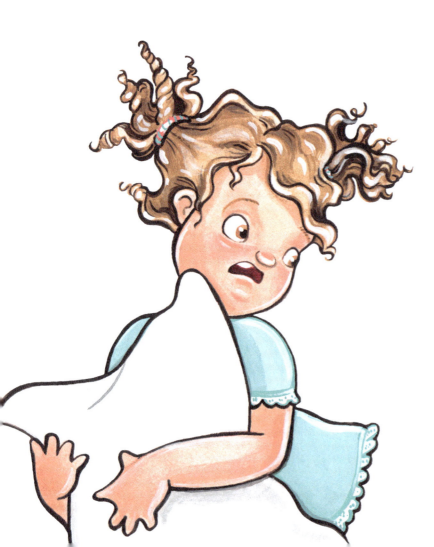
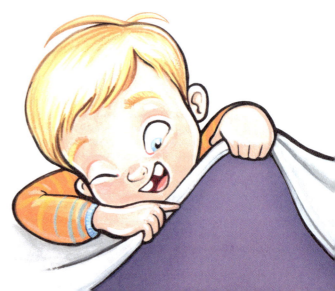

Children asked parents,
their sisters and brothers.
Some asked their neighbors who
even asked others!
All offered answers,
but no one was sure.
And all of their theories were
starting to blur...

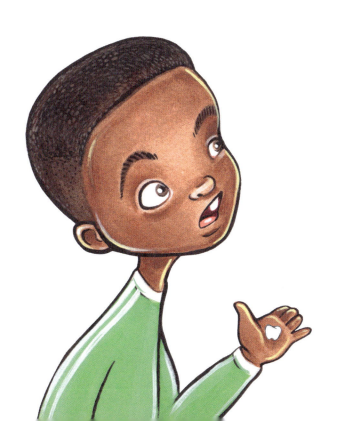
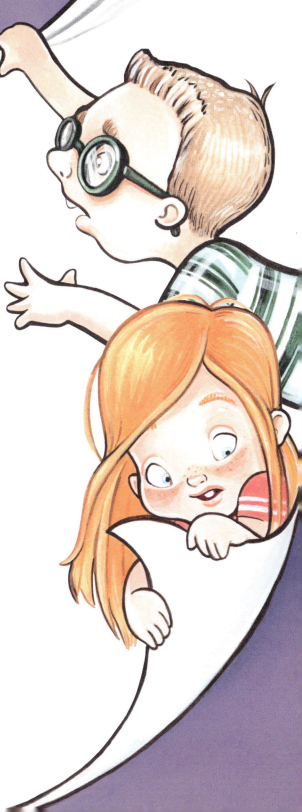

"She forgot."
"She got lost."
"She ran out of money."

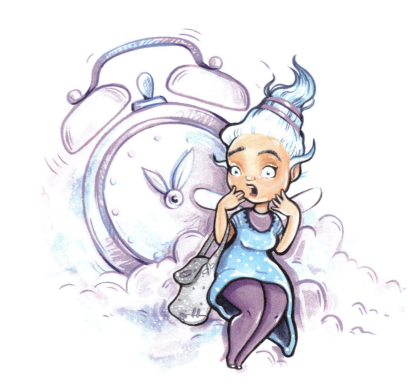
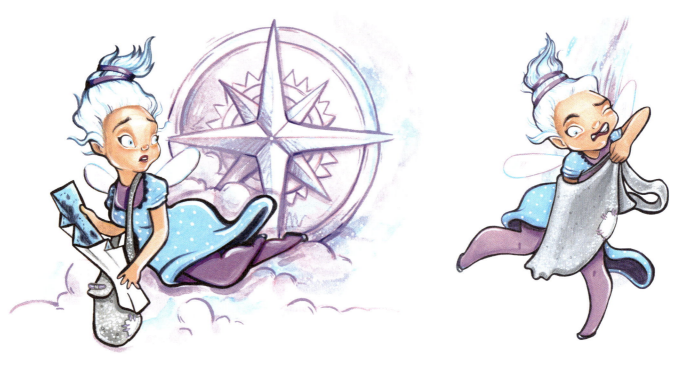

"She went on vacation."
(Now that would be funny.)

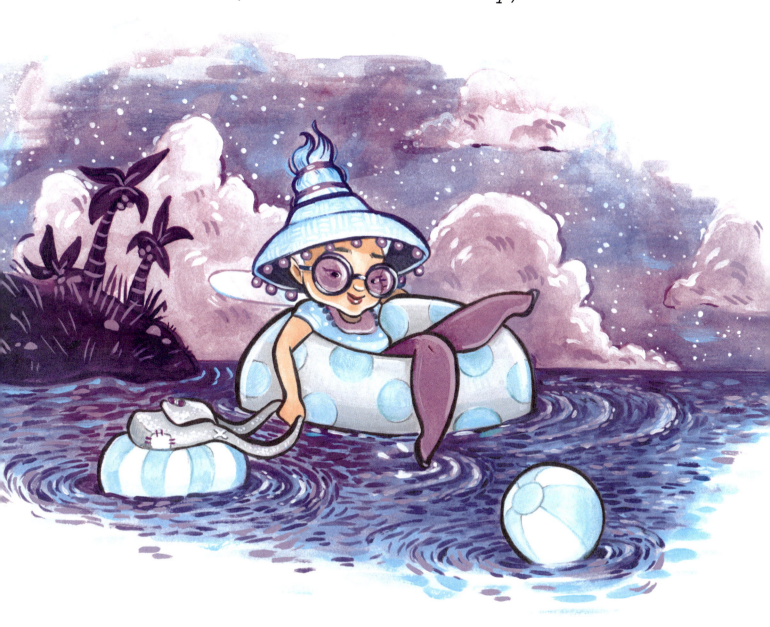

As children grew worried,
a list had grown long,
of theories and what ifs,
but all of them...
WRONG!

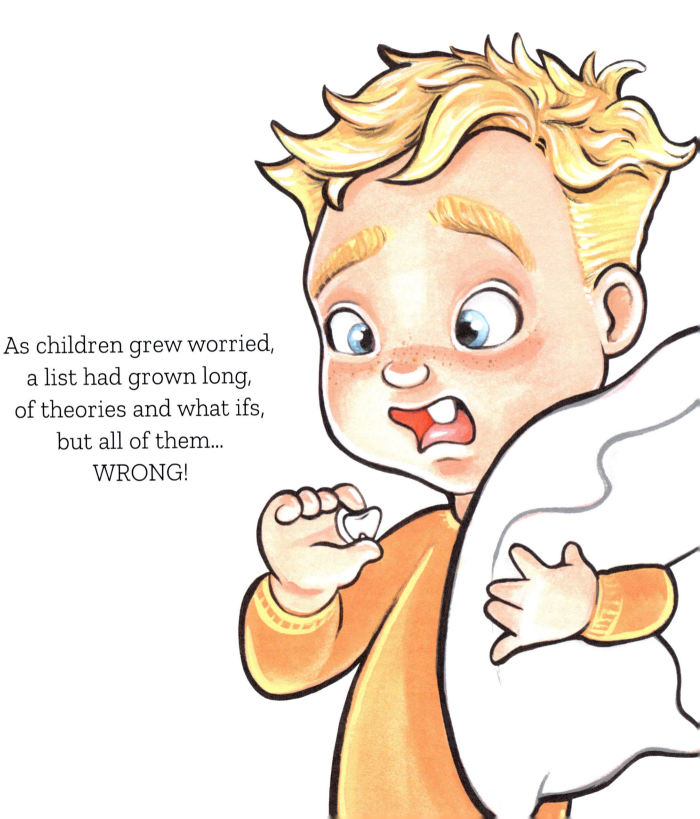

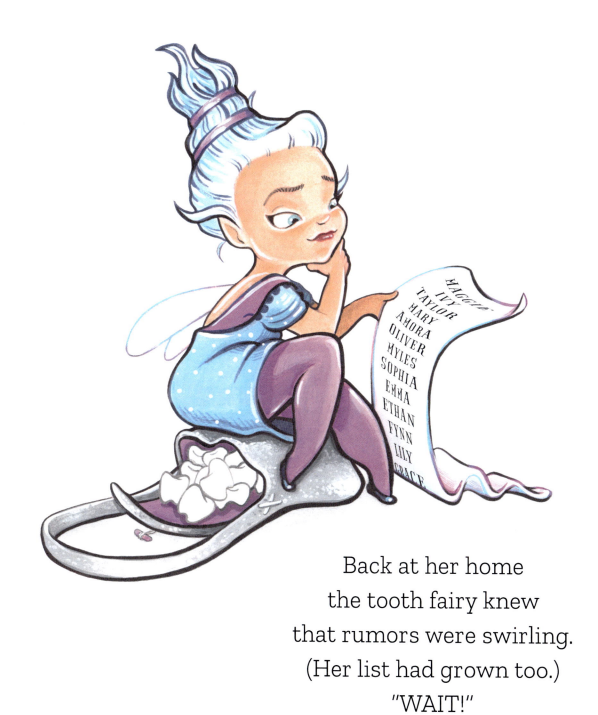

Back at her home
the tooth fairy knew
that rumors were swirling.
(Her list had grown too.)
"WAIT!"

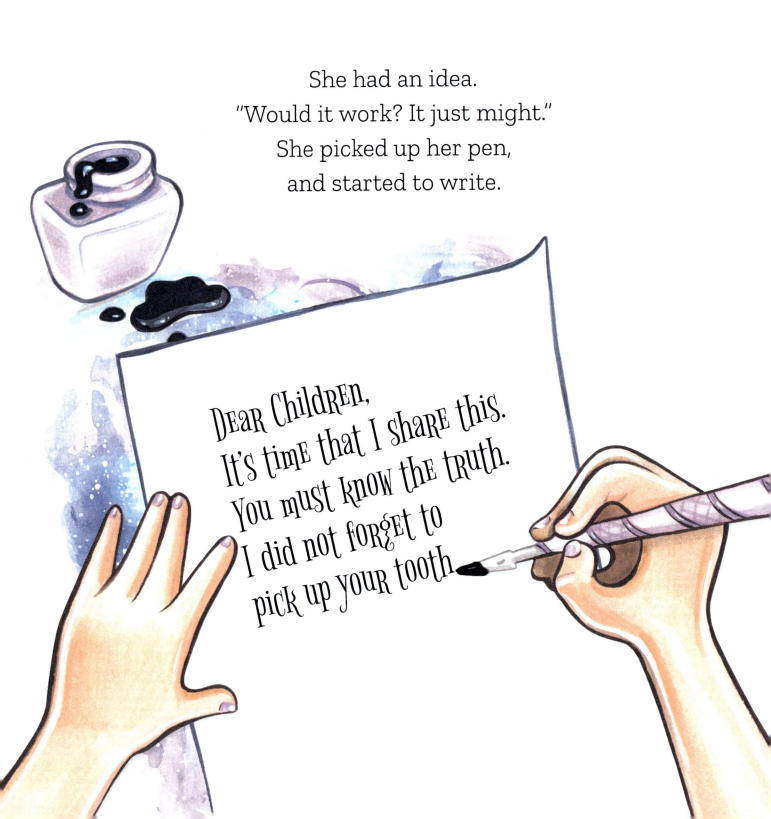

She had an idea.
"Would it work? It just might."
She picked up her pen,
and started to write.

Dear Children,
It's time that I share this.
You must know the truth.
I did not forget to
pick up your tooth

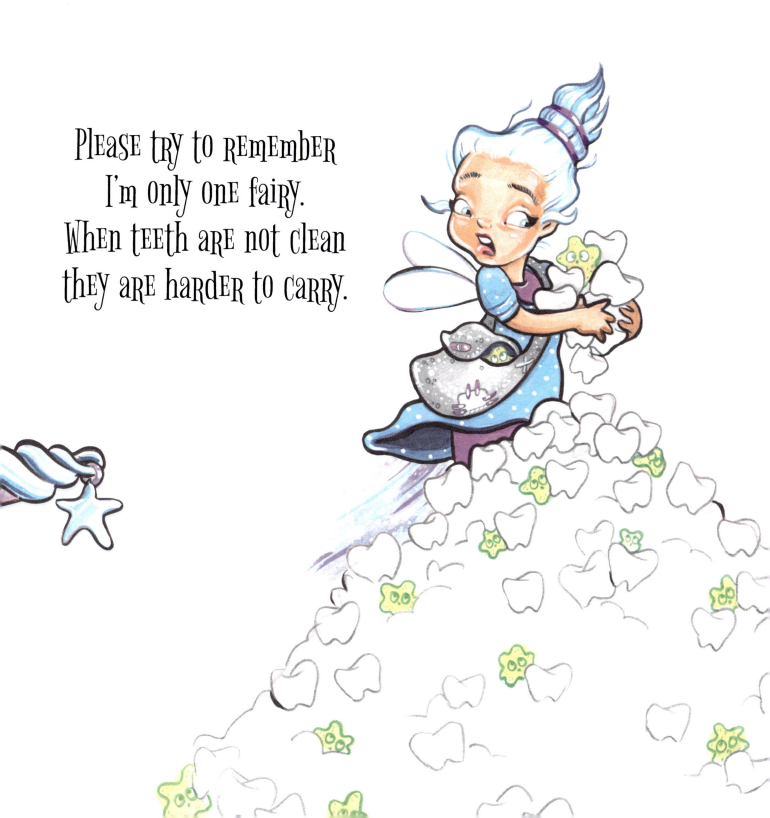

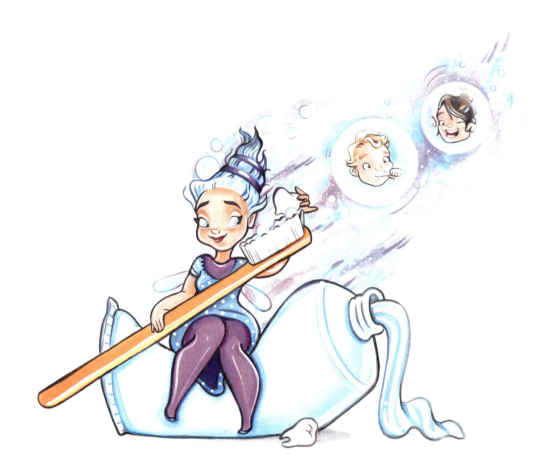

If you are not brushing
to keep your teeth clean
or flossing out food
that sticks in between,
your teeth will weigh more—
Do you know what I mean?

Sugar bugs, plaque and
leftover food,
weigh down my bag.
(I don't mean to be rude.)
And once it's too heavy to
carry and fly,
I must return home
(please excuse the big sigh).

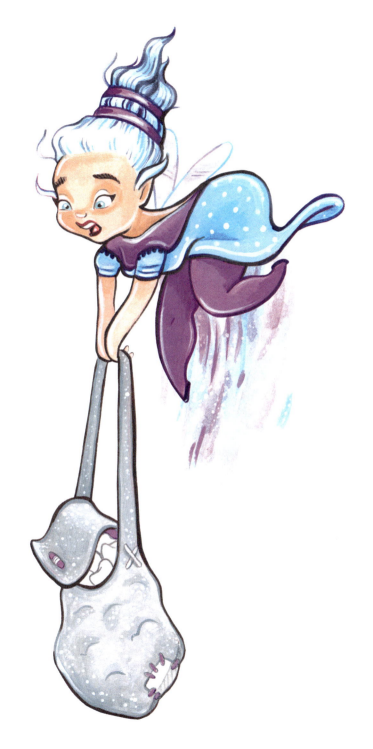

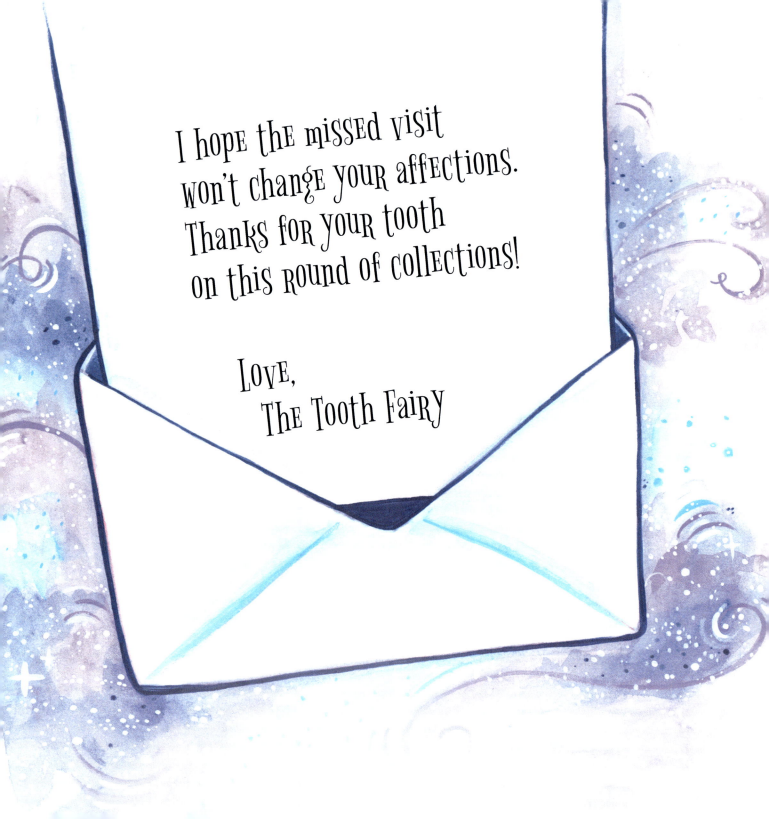

I hope the missed visit
won't change your affections.
Thanks for your tooth
on this round of collections!

Love,
　　The Tooth Fairy

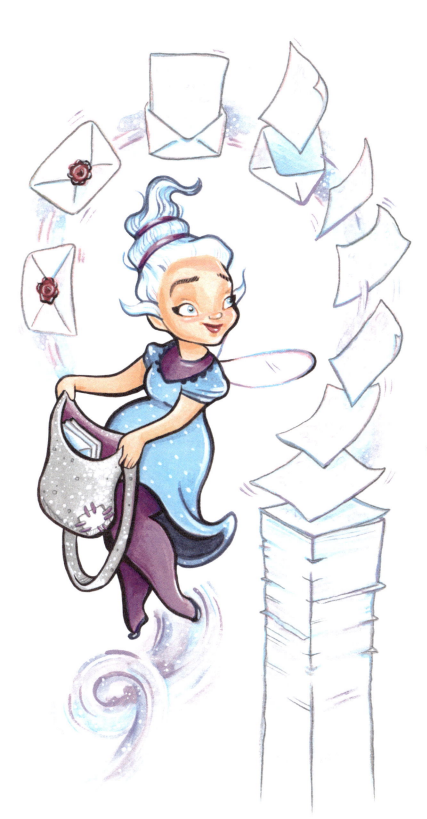

Pleased with her work, she sealed every letter, hopeful their efforts would start to get better. With minutes to spare, she packed her bag tight, then gathered her list and flew into the night.

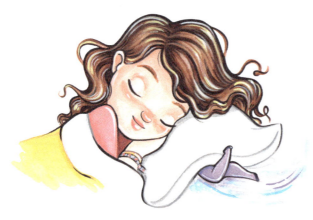

As morning arrived,
children opened their eyes,
and quickly discovered
a special surprise—
their teeth had been taken,
and all was revealed.
Next to their gifts
were the letters she'd sealed.
"The tooth fairy's back!"
They knew what to do.
They'd have to brush better.
They'd need to floss too.

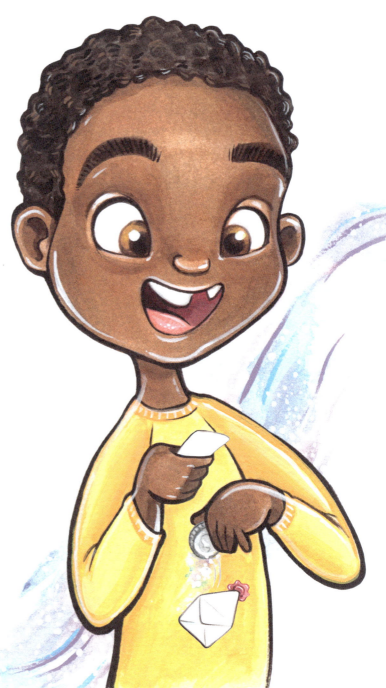

And better they did,
in a wonderful way.
Their wiggly teeth
became cleaner each day.
The children were happy.
Their smiles got brighter.
AND...

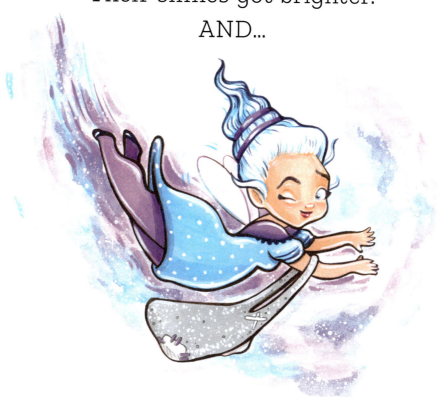

As the tooth fairy hoped,
her bag became lighter!

ACTIVITIES

DRAW IT!

Morning hair don't care!

My cool tooth brush.

My missing tooth smile!

My fav PJ's.

Dental Fun Word Search

BRUSH • FLOSS • SUGAR BUG • GIFT • FAIRY
TOOTH • PLAQUE • LETTER • WIGGLE

F	B	T	O	O	T	H	W
W	R	I	W	B	Q	A	I
S	U	G	A	R	B	U	G
T	S	I	J	W	V	X	G
Q	H	F	L	O	S	S	L
L	E	T	T	E	R	U	E
H	F	A	I	R	Y	R	O
K	N	P	L	A	Q	U	E

CONNECT IT!

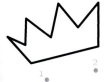
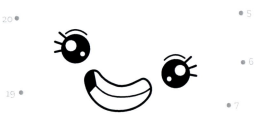

What do you think the tooth fairy does with all those teeth?

Top

Fill in the teeth that already fell out!

Bottom

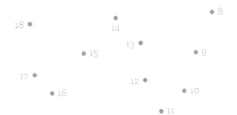

FIND IT!

Find the path that will lead the tooth fairy to the lost tooth.

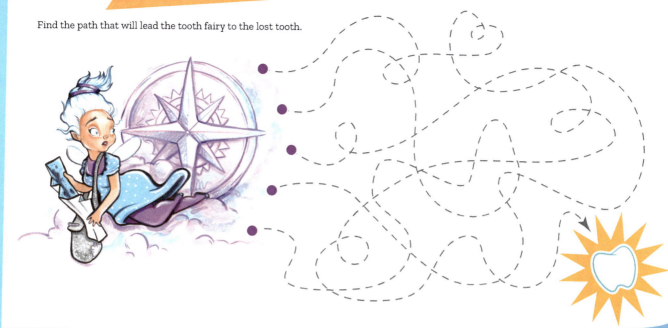

FUN FACTS

How YOU can help the tooth fairy:

When it comes to good brushing, remember the **2 Rule**:
Brush for: 2 minutes, 2 times a day with fluoride toothpaste!

Floss away! Once a day keeps the sugar bugs away.
(Bedtime is the best time.)

Water for the win! Drinking water helps rinse away sugar bugs, plaque, and leftover food. Drink from the sink and you may get the added benefit of fluoride. Find out if your tap water contains fluoride and pour yourself a glass!

Eat up! Whole fruits, whole vegetables, and cheese have something special in common— They all lower your risk of tooth decay.

Following these steps will make your smile brighter!
(And the tooth fairy's bag lighter!)

Fluoride

is a naturally occurring mineral that prevents tooth decay by strengthening tooth enamel.

LOST TOOTH TRACKER

FUN FACT! You will lose 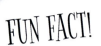 baby teeth!
(Wow! That's a lot of visits from the tooth fairy!)

TOOTH # 1. AGE/DATE LOST: _____ DETAILS: _____ GIFT: _____
TOOTH # 2. AGE/DATE LOST: _____ DETAILS: _____ GIFT: _____
TOOTH # 3. AGE/DATE LOST: _____ DETAILS: _____ GIFT: _____
TOOTH # 4. AGE/DATE LOST: _____ DETAILS: _____ GIFT: _____
TOOTH # 5. AGE/DATE LOST: _____ DETAILS: _____ GIFT: _____
TOOTH # 6. AGE/DATE LOST: _____ DETAILS: _____ GIFT: _____
TOOTH # 7. AGE/DATE LOST: _____ DETAILS: _____ GIFT: _____
TOOTH # 8. AGE/DATE LOST: _____ DETAILS: _____ GIFT: _____
TOOTH # 9. AGE/DATE LOST: _____ DETAILS: _____ GIFT: _____
TOOTH # 10. AGE/DATE LOST: _____ DETAILS: _____ GIFT: _____
TOOTH # 11. AGE/DATE LOST: _____ DETAILS: _____ GIFT: _____
TOOTH # 12. AGE/DATE LOST: _____ DETAILS: _____ GIFT: _____
TOOTH # 13. AGE/DATE LOST: _____ DETAILS: _____ GIFT: _____
TOOTH # 14. AGE/DATE LOST: _____ DETAILS: _____ GIFT: _____
TOOTH # 15. AGE/DATE LOST: _____ DETAILS: _____ GIFT: _____
TOOTH # 16. AGE/DATE LOST: _____ DETAILS: _____ GIFT: _____
TOOTH # 17. AGE/DATE LOST: _____ DETAILS: _____ GIFT: _____
TOOTH # 18. AGE/DATE LOST: _____ DETAILS: _____ GIFT: _____
TOOTH # 19. AGE/DATE LOST: _____ DETAILS: _____ GIFT: _____
TOOTH # 20. AGE/DATE LOST: _____ DETAILS: _____ GIFT: _____

My Brush & Floss Chart

NAME: _____

WEEK 1

	SUNDAY	MONDAY	TUESDAY	WEDNESDAY	THURSDAY	FRIDAY	SATURDAY
☀							
🌙							
🌙							

WEEK 2

	SUNDAY	MONDAY	TUESDAY	WEDNESDAY	THURSDAY	FRIDAY	SATURDAY
☀							
🌙							
🌙							

My Brush & Floss Chart

NAME: _____

	SUNDAY	MONDAY	TUESDAY	WEDNESDAY	THURSDAY	FRIDAY	SATURDAY
WEEK 3							

	SUNDAY	MONDAY	TUESDAY	WEDNESDAY	THURSDAY	FRIDAY	SATURDAY
WEEK 4							

Made in the USA
Middletown, DE
18 April 2023